Yoga For Weight Loss

Discover How To Use Yoga to Lose Weight, Burn Fat and Stay Slim and Young.

By Gary Jay

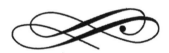

Copyright 2015. All rights reserved.

This document is geared towards providing exact and reliable information in regards to the topic and issue covered. The publication is sold with the idea that the publisher is not required to render accounting, officially permitted, or otherwise, qualified services. If advice is necessary, legal or professional, a practiced individual in the profession should be ordered.

- From a Declaration of Principles which was accepted and approved equally by a Committee of the American Bar Association and a Committee of Publishers and Associations.

In no way is it legal to reproduce, duplicate, or transmit any part of this document in either electronic means or in printed format. Recording of this publication is strictly prohibited and any storage of this document is not allowed unless with written permission from the publisher. All rights reserved.

The information provided herein is stated to be truthful and consistent, in that any liability, in terms of inattention or otherwise, by any usage or abuse of any policies, processes, or directions contained within is the solitary and utter responsibility of the recipient reader. Under no circumstances will any legal responsibility or blame be held against the publisher for any reparation, damages, or monetary loss due to the information herein, either directly or indirectly.

Respective authors own all copyrights not held by the publisher.

The information herein is offered for informational purposes solely, and is universal as so. The presentation of the information is without contract or any type of guarantee assurance.

The trademarks that are used are without any consent, and the publication of the trademark is without permission or backing by the trademark owner. All trademarks and brands within this book are for clarifying purposes only and are the owned by the owners themselves, not affiliated with this document.

Table of Contents

Introduction

Yoga: A brief Overview

Yoga for weight loss

Yoga poses for Weight loss

1. The Warrior Pose
2. The Half Moon Pose
3. The Tree Pose
4. The Half Spinal Twist
5. The Cobbler Pose
6. The Chair Pose
7. The Bridge Pose
8. The Downward Dog Pose
9. The Side Plank Pose
10. The Half Wheel Pose
11. The Cobra pose

BONUS: Weight Loss Dieting

Important Note

Conclusion

Introduction

I want to thank you and congratulate you for buying the book, *"Yoga For Weight loss: Discover How To Use Yoga to Lose Weight, Burn Fat and Stay Slim and Young"*.

This book has actionable information on how to use yoga for weight loss and relaxation.

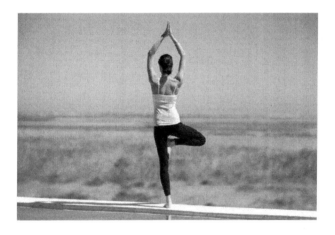

Yoga is a technique that can get you to overcome many of the problems that you've been struggling with for years. It is not just about doing some crazy and seemingly impossible poses that makes yoga great; it has a lot more benefits that you can derive through consistent practice including weight loss, relaxation, stress relief and fostering inner peace, which is a rare commodity in our current generation. If you want to learn how to make this possible, this book will help you to unleash the full power of yoga to your advantage.

Thanks again for buying this book, I hope you enjoy it!

Yoga: A Brief Overview

What is It?

For starters, yoga is more than doing some seemingly impossible and pretty weird twisted poses. Yoga is derived from the Sankrit word "yuj", which "to integrate or to unite". It entails harmonizing the mind with the body and breath through different breathing techniques, yoga poses (referred to as asanas) and meditation.

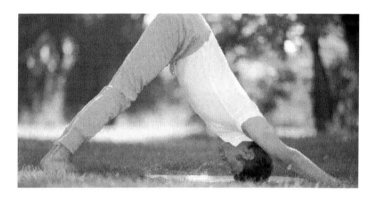

Yoga is a mental, physical, and spiritual practice, which can be practiced for various reasons. This ancient art originated from India, and it is based on harmonizing the development system of the mind, body and spirit. Its ultimate goal is liberation, which is why the continued practice of yoga will lead to a sense of peace and well-being.

Practicing yoga brings about emotional stability and clarity of your mind. It also improves the functionality of the digestive, hormonal, circulative and the respiratory systems besides making your body strong and flexible.

Yoga for Weight Loss

I know that if you are new to yoga, the last thing you would have thought that the poses can do for you is lose weight. We've somehow been conditioned to believe that for us to lose weight through physical activity, we have to spend endless hours at the gym lifting weights. Well, while the simple formula for weight loss is that you must create a calorie deficit by burning more calories than you've consumed (something which even the most strenuous yoga pose may not achieve unless you do it for several hours), the truth is that yoga does help in weight loss. So if burning calories is not the reason why you are likely to lose weight, what does cause weight loss when you do yoga?

So how does yoga do it?

Well, simple; yoga does it in 2 broad ways:

1. Yoga helps you to combat stress thus reducing the likelihood of you eating to cope with stress

2. Yoga can help you with mindful eating and mindfulness, which are all essential in coping with stress and helping you to notice when you've had enough food thus reducing the chances of overeating due to mindless eating. Yoga helps to increase body awareness especially on matters pertaining hunger and satiety, which makes it pretty easy for you to lose weight in the process.

3. Yoga can improve blood circulation throughout the body, which facilitates in increasing your flexibility, energy level and loosing excess unwanted fat content.

4. Yoga improves your resistance to diseases, as the poses and movements in

yoga massage the internal organs, which improves their functionality.

As you can see, with yoga, it is possible to melt fat away without breaking too much sweat. Well, for starters always associate weight loss with heavy physical exercises and dieting without paying attention to our spiritual and emotional needs. In other words, we do not address the root issue as to why you could be overeating or having a problem shedding those extra pounds due to high stress levels.

The truth is that weight loss needs to be addressed with spiritual and emotional means because it is a spiritual and emotional problem. Yoga stimulates and fulfills you emotionally, mentally, physically, and spiritually. Your sense of self-worth is improved when you feel fulfilled on all levels. With increased self-love and self-esteem, you will begin to lose weight naturally since you will not have to overeat as a way of getting back to yourself, as you could have done before.

In simple terms, you benefit from yoga through mindfulness and stress reduction, all of which can help you have better eating habits, better sleep, and greater self-awareness. All these have a role to play in helping you to lose and maintain weight loss over time.

If you practice the right form of yoga, it is a great way to lose weight because it is light on your joints and has minimum chances of injury. You don't have to go to the gym to practice it; you can always do it at the comfort of your home. All you need is a Yoga mat and some comfortable clothes. Let's take a quick look at some of the poses you can do to help you lose weight.

Yoga Poses for Weight Loss

The Warrior Pose

Besides helping you lose weight, this pose will be of benefit to your tummy, buttocks and thighs given that it helps strengthen them.

How to do it

1. Stand with hands by your side and your feet together.

2. Extend you left foot backwards and your right foot forward.

3. Bend your right knee to ensure you get into a lunge position.

4. Twist your torso to face away from right knee that is bent.

5. Turn your left foot at an angle of about 4o degrees sideways so that you can get the right support.

6. Inhale as you raise your body up and away from your knee that is bent. Straighten your arms.

7. Stretch the arms upwards and turn your torso slowly backward so that your back forms an arch.

8. Exhale and straighten your right knee to get out of this pose. Push off your right leg and come back to your original position. Do not rush out of it to avoid any injury. Repeat this procedure for the other leg.

    Tips and Precaution: Avoid bending the pelvis forward. People with neck pain, do not strain.

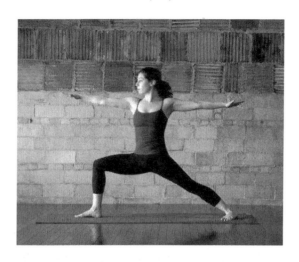

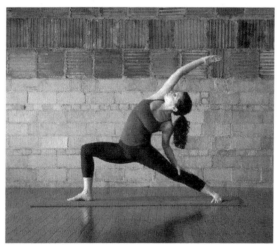

The Warrior Pose

The Half Moon Pose

This pose helps you to burn off the love handles and strengthen your core. It also tones your inner and upper thighs and buttocks.

How to do it:

1. Stand straight with your feet together.
2. Clasp your palms together after raising your hands above your head. Extend the stretch by trying to reach the ceiling.
3. Exhale and bend sideways slowly from your hips. Keep your elbows straight and do not bend forward. You should feel a stretch from your thighs to your fingertips.
4. Inhale and come back to your original position. Repeat this for the other leg.

    Tips and Precaution: If you find difficulty touching the floor, use a block. Do not strain your arms and neck.

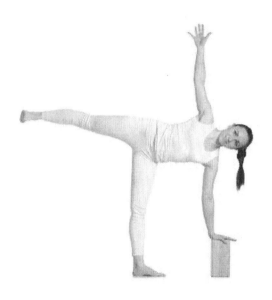

The Half Moon Pose

The Tree Pose

This pose is great for your abdominal muscles. It also tones your arms and thighs.

How to do it:

1. Stand with your legs together.

2. Put most of your weight on your right leg and just a little on the other.

3. Raise your left leg so that it faces inwards towards your right leg.

4. Place the heel of your foot on your inner thigh of the other leg, as close to the pelvis as possible.

5. Gently raise your arms above your head ensuring your fingers point towards the ceiling.

6. Focus your mind on one spot and breathe steadily to maintain your balance.

Tips and Precaution: Keep the eyes open initially. Once you can get 'locked; in position, close your eyes.

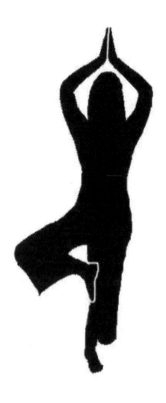

The Tree Pose

The Half-Spinal Twist

This pose stimulates your digestive system thus helping you to digest food more efficiently and lose weight. It stretches your spine and tones your thighs and the muscles of the abdomen.

How to do it

1. Sit up with your legs stretched out right in front of you. Keep your spine erect and your feet together.

2. Bend your left leg and place the heel of your left foot beside your right hip.

3. Take the right leg over your left knee and place your left hand on your right knee and your right hand behind you.

4. Twist at the waist, shoulders and neck in that sequence to the right and look over the right shoulder.

5. Hold and continue with long and gentle breaths, breathing in and out.

6. Come back to your starting position and continue breathing out. Release your right foot first, then the waist, then the chest and finally the neck. Then sit up relaxed but still straight.

7. Repeat this procedure from the other side.

Tips and Precaution: Do not lean the body drop the shoulders or lift buttocks of the ground. Avoid this exercise if you have severe back pain.

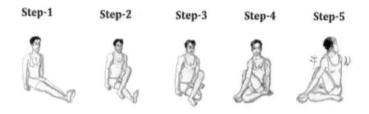

The Half-Spinal Twist

The Cobbler Pose

Besides relieving menstrual discomfort and improving on your digestion, this pose helps to reduce the fat on your inner thighs and usually strengthens your spine, knees, muscles of the groin and lower back.

How to do it

1. Sit on your mat stretching your legs right in front of you.

2. Bend your legs at your knees making sure that your spine erect. The soles of your feet should face each other.

3. Use your hands to pull your legs in so that your legs touch each other. Make them to be as close to the pelvis as possible.

4. Move your thighs up and down while holding your legs at the ankles. Do this as many times as you can.

Tips and Precaution: Avoid fast jerky movements. Avoid this pose if you have hip or shoulder injury.

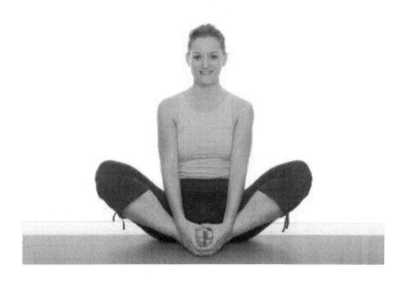

The Cobbler Pose

The Chair Pose

This yoga pose helps in strengthening the thighs, abdomen, spine and buttocks.

How to do it

1. Begin by standing straight.

2. Stretch hands up in the air (feel the stretch).

3. Bend your knees slowly and come down, until, the thighs are parallel to the ground.

4. Stay in this position for 30 seconds and come back to the starting position.

    Tips and Precaution: Practice the pose near a wall to maintain balance. Avoid this pose if you feel dizziness.

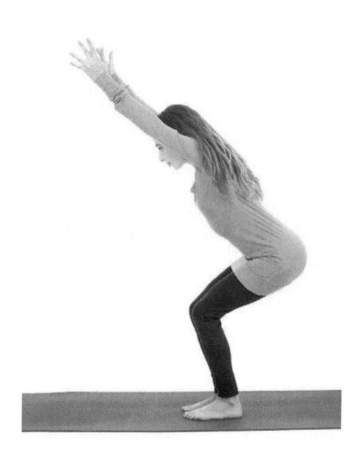

The Chair Pose

The Bridge Pose

1. Lie on your back. Bend the knees, placing the feet flat on the floor, 1 foot apart. Keep the arms alongside the body with the palms facing down.

2. Press the feet firmly on the floor. Inhale and lift the hips up, rolling the spine off the floor.

3. Lightly squeeze the knees together to keep the feet, 1 foot apart.

4. Press down into the arms and shoulders and lift the chest up. Lift the hips higher, by engaging the legs and buttocks.

5. Breathe and hold for 30 seconds.

6. Exhale and slowly roll the spine back to the floor and the feet straight and relaxed.

Tips and Precaution: Avoid this pose if you have neck pain, back pain, hip pain or shoulder pain.

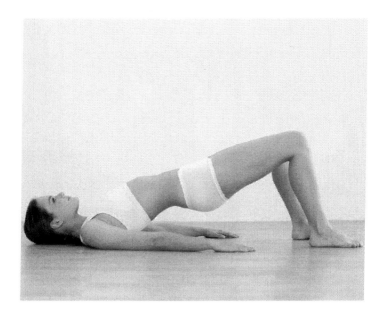

The Bridge Pose

The Downward facing Dog Pose

This yoga pose will improve digestion and provides relief from back pain and fatigue. It energizes the body, by improving blood circulation and would also calm the mind as well as relieve stress.

How to do it

1. Come down forward, bending your hip and try to touch the ground (bend knees if required).

2. Keep your palms firmly on the ground and step back (one foot at a time).

3. Hold the position for 30 seconds, while, breathing calmly.

4. Come back to the normal position and repeat the process the 5 times.

   Tips and Precaution: Initially try keeping hands on a chair or block. Do not do this pose if you have migraine or high blood pressure.

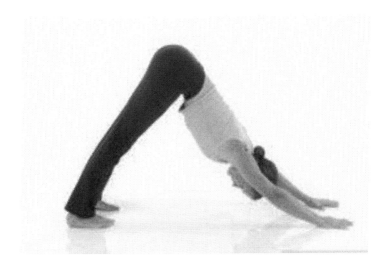

The Downward facing Dog Pose

The Side Plank Pose

This yoga pose helps in stretching the arms, belly and legs and will also improve the balance.

How to do it

1. Begin from the downward facing dog pose
2. Keep your feet together and press your body weight down the right hand and forearm.
3. Twist your body to the right and balance on your feet and right hand.
4. Align your body in a straight line.
5. Extend your left hand straight up, towards the sky. Look up, at your left hand.
6. Exhale slowly and come back to the downward dog pose.

Tips and Precaution: Try this pose with the help of a support or a wall. Do not do this pose if you are not completely fit.

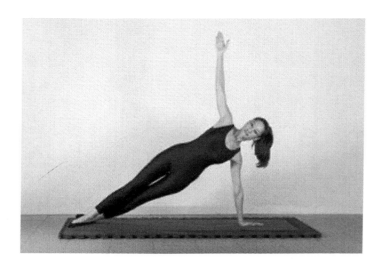

The Side Plank Pose

The Half Wheel Pose

This yoga pose stimulates abdominal organs and aids in digestion. It is also very effective in treating lower back pain and reducing belly fat.

How to do it

1. Stand up straight. Keep your feet close together and arms alongside your body.

2. Inhale and extend your arms (pivoting at the shoulder) over your head and keeping your palms facing each other.

3. Bend backwards, as you push your hip forward and keep your arms in line with your ears. Keep your elbows and knees straight and look up.

4. Keep your chest, facing the ceiling.

5. Hold the pose for 15 seconds. Slowly come back up, exhaling.

Tips and Precaution: Avoid this if you have hip or spinal problem.

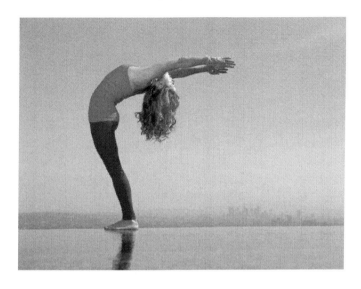

The Half Wheel Pose

The Cobra Pose

This Yoga pose is one of the simplest but the most effective. It stimulates the abdominal muscles and organs. It stretches the chest, providing relief from stress. This technique is known to produce body heat and burn fat.

How to do it

1. Lie flat on the ground, with your forehead touching the ground. Relax.
2. Place your palms (face down), below the shoulders and close to the body.
3. Slowly Inhale and straighten your arms and lift your chest up, till the upper body is raised into a curve. Look up.
4. Keep the legs firmly on the ground and this position for 30 seconds (breathe slowly) and come back down slowly, exhaling.

   Tips and Precaution: Do not do this pose if you have serious back/ spinal problem.

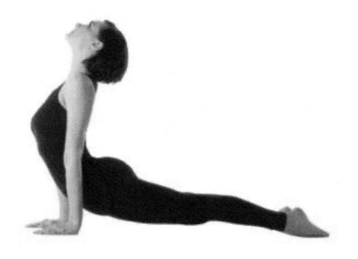

The Cobra Pose

BONUS: Weight Loss Dieting tips

Keep the Weight Off

There is no easy way to lose weight. Losing weight is not about eating less, but eating SMART. According to experts, the only way to shed excess weight is to burn more calories than you eat.

60 % Americans are overweight and spend $25 billion dollar each year for different weight loss programs. But I will tell you the secret. It's all in the determination and the will power you have. You can spend all the money you have, but if you don't have the will power to make the change and follow it, nothing's going to happen. If you are reading this, then follow it.

Focus on long term. A diet that is high in meat and low in fruits may lead to short term weight loss. When people want to lose weight, they want instant results. Experts suggest a goal of losing 1lb (3500 calories) a week is healthy. Therefore reduce food intake by 500 calories a day. Or eat 250 fewer calories and burn 250 more through exercise.

What you need to know before dieting...

NEVER skip your Breakfast: Do not start of the day with an empty stomach. Researchers have discovered a hormone called ghrelin, secreted by the stomach and its level rises with an empty stomach, which makes you to run for any food.

CARBS are important: Do not believe the myth. You need carbohydrates. Just sty away from simple carbs, like sugar, white bread, white pasta and white rice. These foods increase the level of glucose in our body; not good for weight loss.

Start eating more complex carb food, like whole-grain, vegetables, and fruits. Have more lean meat, white beans, egg white, mashed potatoes and corn flakes.

Eat food rich in high fiber: These foods don't leave you hungry. Some examples are- Lentils, black beans, broccolis, raspberries, blackberries, pears, bran flakes.

AVOID low fat-foods: That includes dairy products, sausages, bacon and cold cuts. Replace the meat you eat with fish. Avoid fast foods.

Drink plenty of water: Fluids help in quenching thirst and also reduce your appetite. Fruit juices are healthy, but they add calories without fiber. Coffee or tea is fine but not replacement water. Be aware that a glass of wine or beer as 100 calories in it.

Never fast: Weight loss during fasting is not long term. Fasting, even when plenty of water is consumed is dangerous. It can lead to low blood pressure and heart failure.

10 most important weigh loss foods...

1. Whole eggs: They are high in protein, healthy fat and makes you feel full with low calories.
2. Leafy Greens: like kale, spinach, collards, Swiss chards. They are low in calories but high in fiber content.
3. Salmon and tuna: High in Omega 3-fatty acid (helps in beating obesity) and high quality protein.
4. Lean meat: high in protein.
5. Cruciferous vegetables: Like broccoli, cauliflower, cabbage and Brussels sprouts heave a perfect combination of protein and fiber; important for weight loss.
6. Boiled potatoes: including sweet potatoes, turnips and other root vegetables. They are high in resistant starch (a fiber like content)
7. Beans and legumes: High in protein and fiber.
8. Fruits; especially avocados.

9. Coconut oil and extra virgin oil: best source of healthy fat.
10. Some whole grain: like brown rice, oats, quinoas

Important note:

While yoga can help you shed pounds effortlessly, the truth is that it is not a magic wand that you pull when you want to fit into your dinner dress; you have to be careful with your diet to see the results you want to see so badly. In other words, you have to combine proper exercise with eating right.

Eat Healthy, Work Healthy and Stay Healthy.

Make sure to focus on your breathing, while doing each routine. That is the **KEY**, to produce maximum result, fast.

Take help from someone. Feel free, to take assistance, if you find the routines to be tough to execute, by yourself.

Conclusion

Every time you attend a yoga session, you come out as a different person from the person you were before you started. Yoga will give you a relief from countless ailments both at the physical and spiritual level. Work on this art passionately and you will see the results.

Thank you again for buying this book!

I hope this book was able to help you to understand how to use yoga for weight loss, relaxation, inner peace, mindfulness and a lot more.

The next step is to implement what you've just learnt.

Thank you and good luck!

Gary Jay

Made in the USA
San Bernardino, CA
30 October 2018